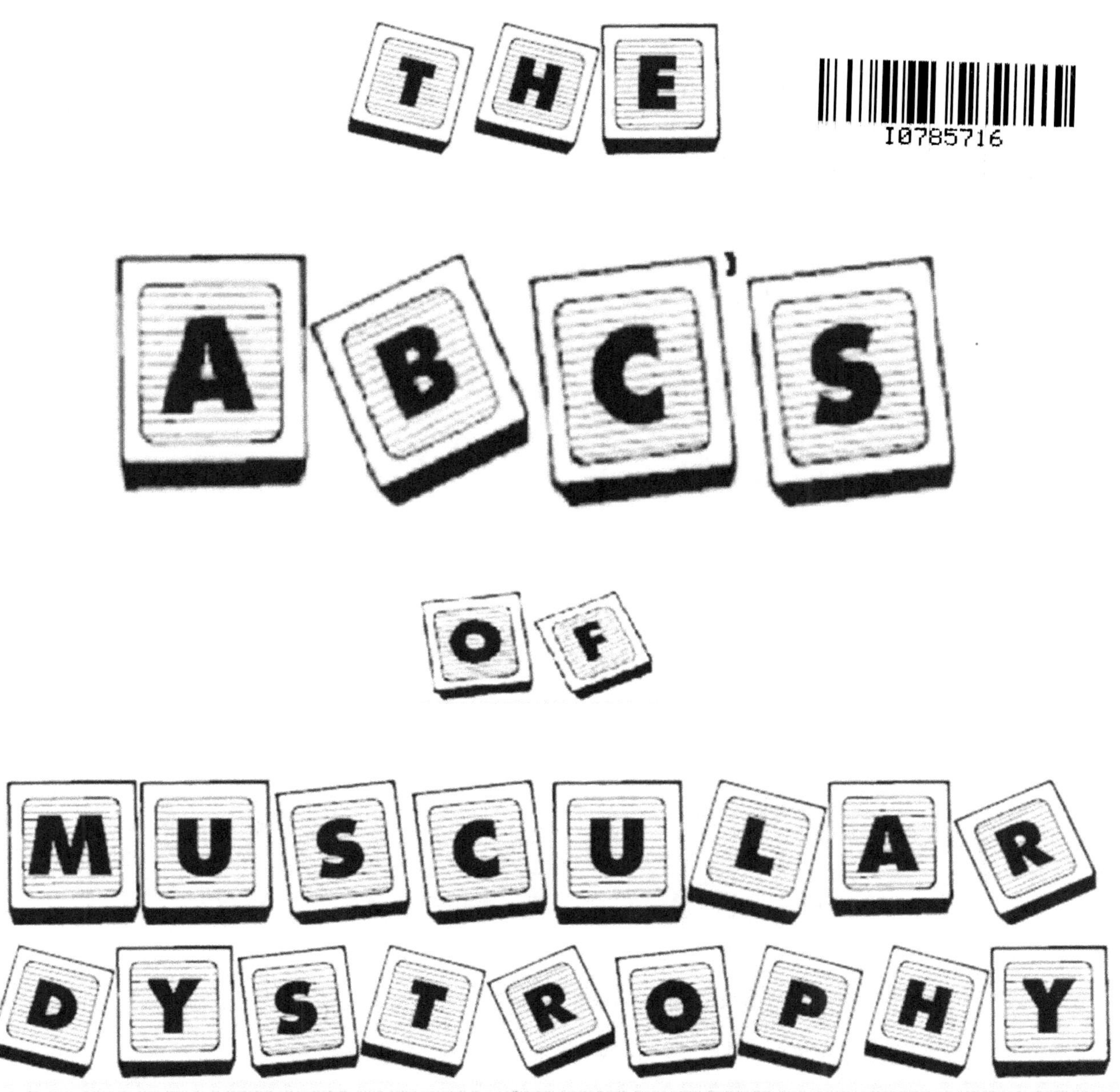

Written By: Melissa Farrell

ISBN: 1723240737
ISBN-13: 978-1723240737

For Frank...

You could have done so much more,
if you only had time.

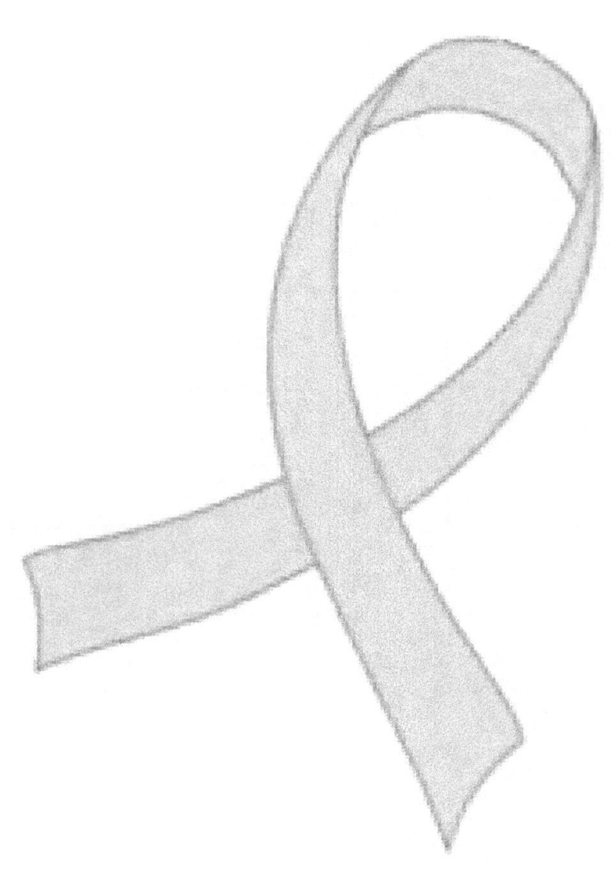

A is for ALS

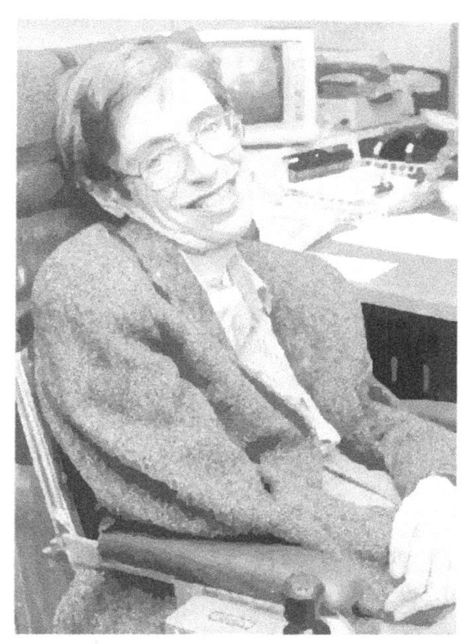

British scientist, Stephen Hawking,
lived with ALS for 55 years.

ALS is a motor neuron disease that affects the nerve cells that control voluntary muscle movement, like walking and talking. ALS is also known as Lou Gehrig's Disease, named after the famous baseball player who was diagnosed with it in 1939.

B is for Becker

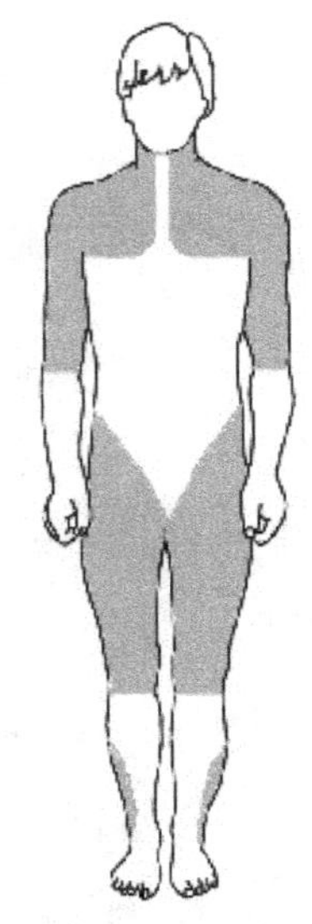

Muscle weakness occurs mostly in the arms, legs, and pelvis.

Becker Muscular Dystrophy is very similar to Duchenne MD. The main difference is that it gets worse at a much slower rate and it is less common. Becker MD is inherited and passed down through families. Becker MD occurs in about 3 to 6 of every 100,000 births. This disease is found mostly in boys.

C is for Congenital

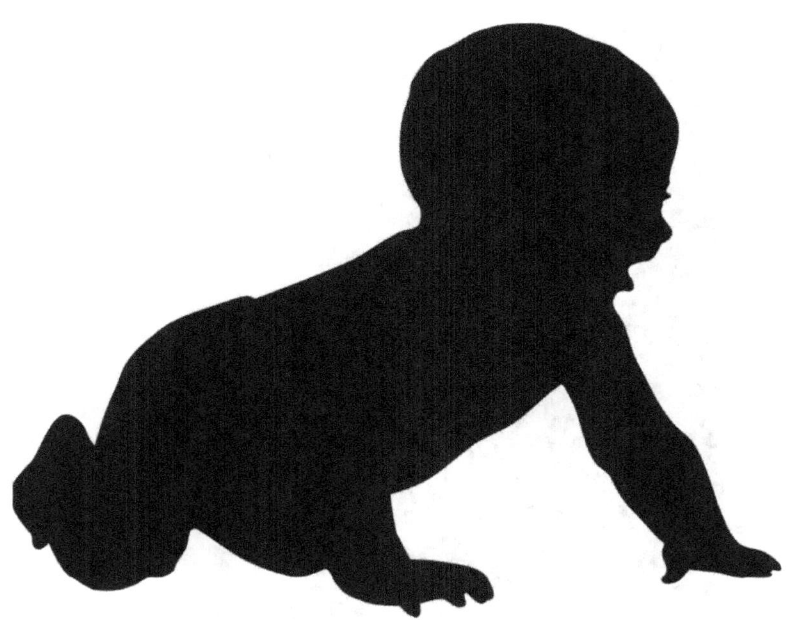

Congenital Muscular Dystrophy is a group of genetic muscle diseases that occur at birth or during infancy. Babies are weak and may have difficulty breathing or swallowing. These infants and toddlers may have trouble rolling over, sitting up, and learning to walk.

D is for Duchenne

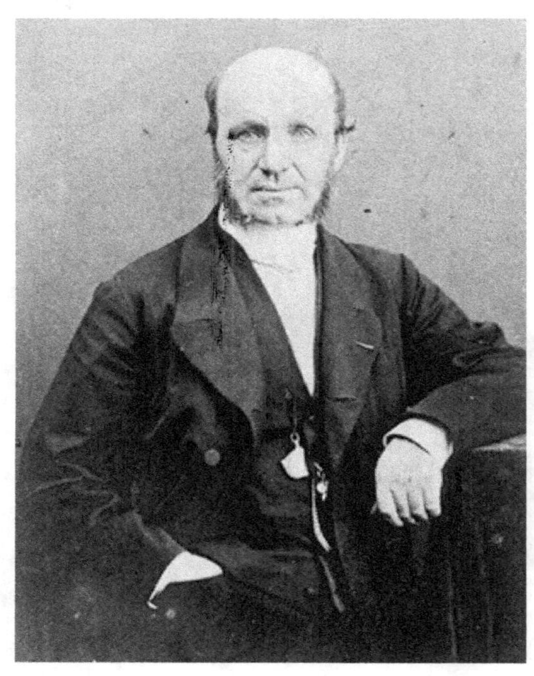

Duchenne de Boulogne was the first to describe the disease
now known as Duchenne Muscular Dystrophy.

Duchenne Muscular Dystrophy is the most common type of MD. It is also the most severe. It affects about 1 out of every 3,500 boys. Children with Duchenne MD may have trouble walking, running, and climbing stairs. Most children require a wheelchair by the age of 13.

E is for Exercise

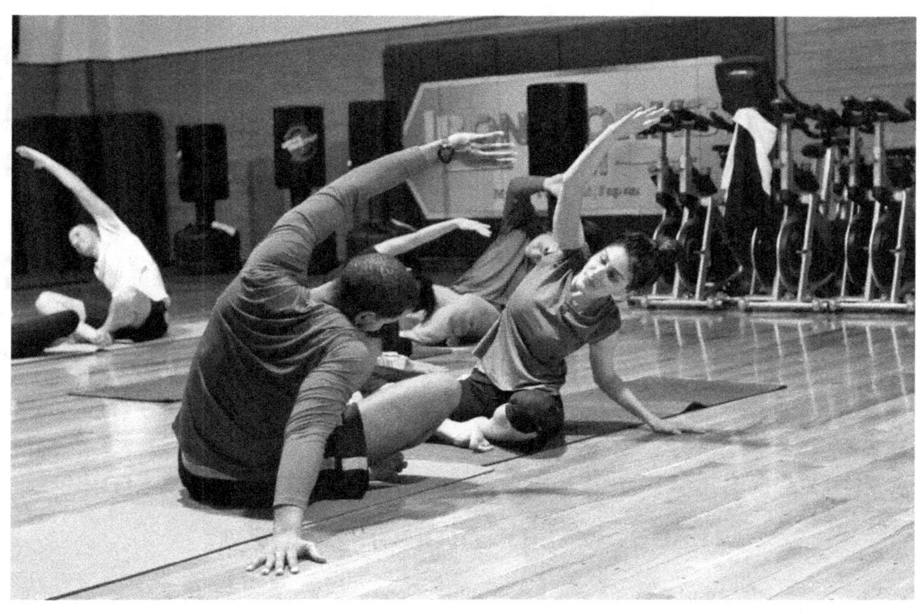

Exercises can help people with muscular dystrophy to keep their muscles flexible and strong. Stretching can help with joint flexibility. Physical therapists will teach activities to promote muscle strength. Too much exercise can have a negative effect. Breathing exercises for respiratory strength are also important.

F is for FSHD

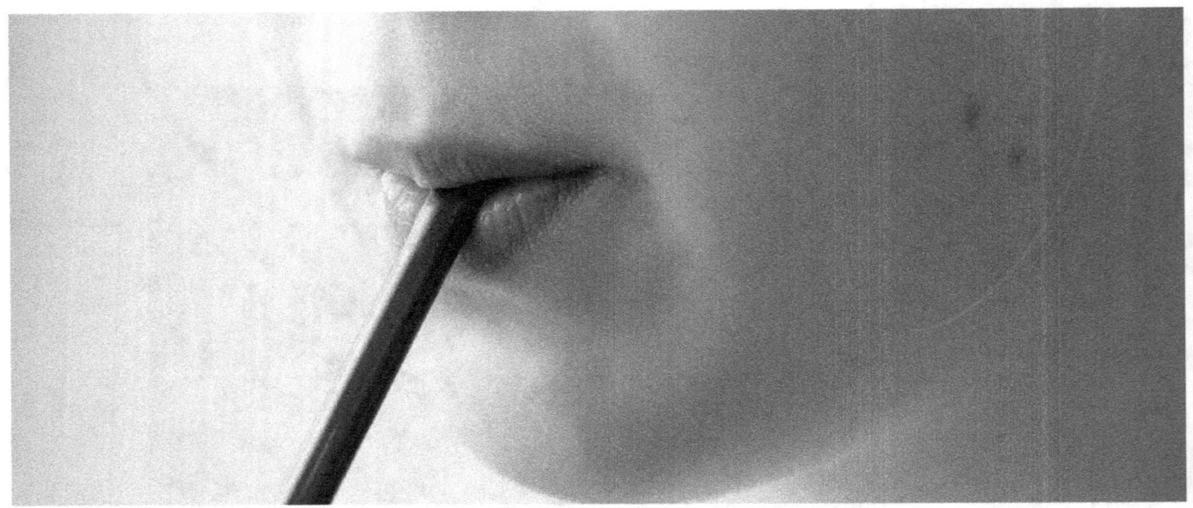

Symptoms of FSHD include the inability to smile,
whistle, or sip through a straw.

Facioscapulohumeral Muscular Dystrophy (**FSHD**)

-affects boys and girls equally

-symptoms begin to appear in the teen years

-muscles in the upper arms, shoulder blades, and face are often the most affected

-also causes weakness in other muscles

G is for Genetic

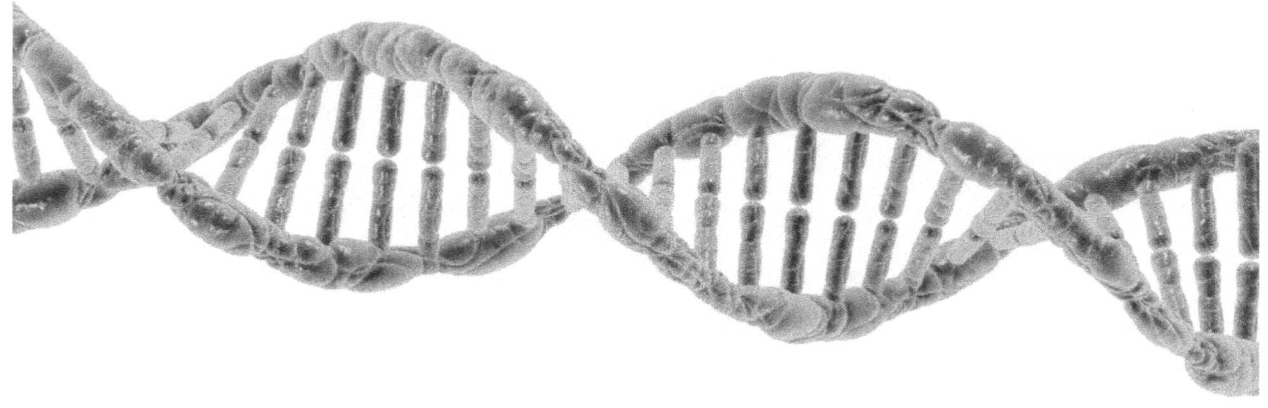

Muscular Dystrophy is not a disease that you can catch from someone else. It is a **genetic** disorder. That means that you inherit the genes when you are born. In most cases, muscular dystrophy runs in families. People with muscular dystrophy do not have the correct information in their genes. This prevents their body from making the proteins that it needs for healthy muscles.

H is for Heart

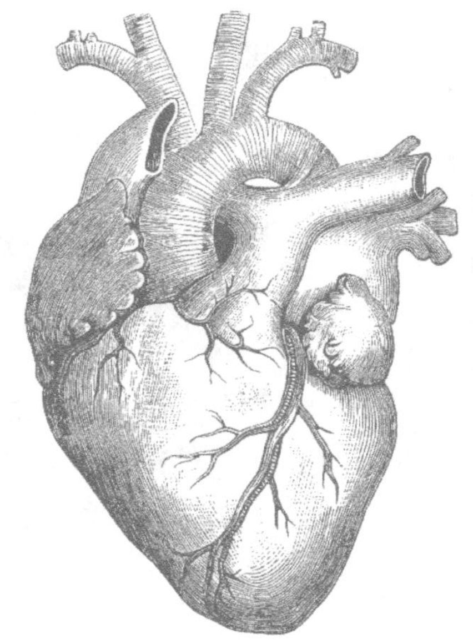

Muscular Dystrophy affects your muscles, and your **heart** is a muscle too! Heart issues may include:

-heart muscle weakness

-heart not pumping blood properly

-arrhythmia: heart beats in an abnormal rhythm

-tachycardia: heart rate is too fast

-bradychardia: heart rate is too slow

I is for Impact

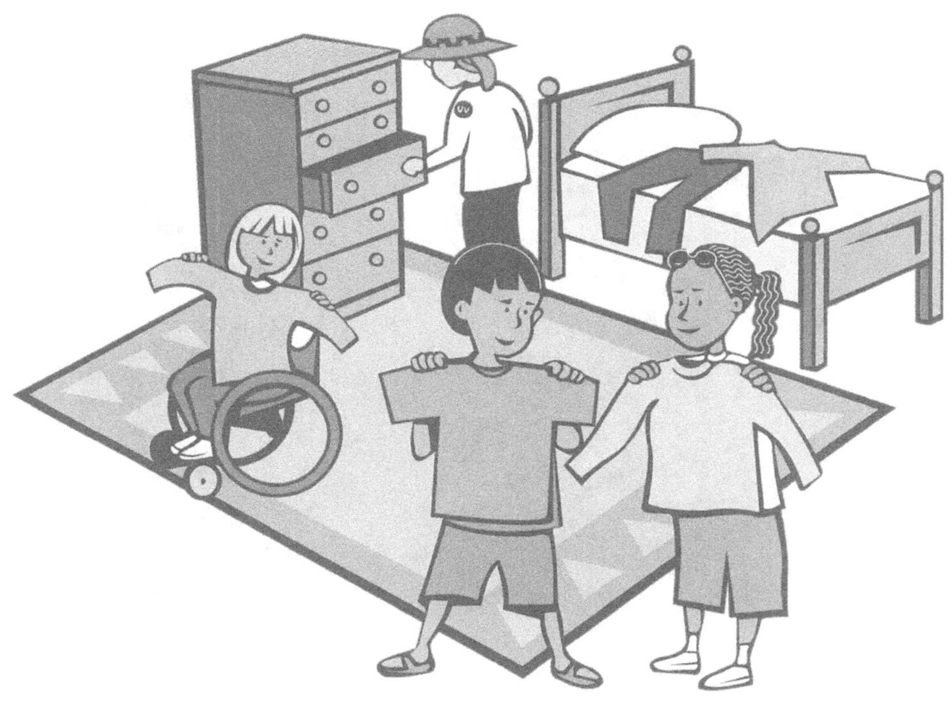

Muscular Dystrophy can **impact** a person's ability to:

-get dressed	-walk and run
-use the stairs	-eat and drink
-write	-complete school work
-balance	-play sports

J is for Jerry Lewis

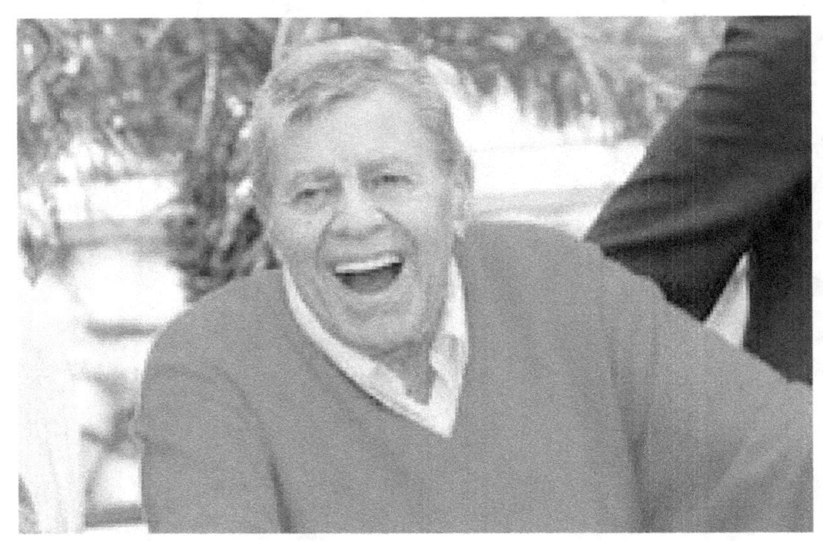

Jerry Lewis was a comedian who was famous for hosting the Labor Day Muscular Dystrophy telethon on TV. Over 45 years, Jerry Lewis raised over $2 billion for muscular dystrophy. In 1977, Jerry Lewis was nominated for a Nobel Peace Prize for his work for the Muscular Dystrophy Association.

K is for WAL<u>K</u>

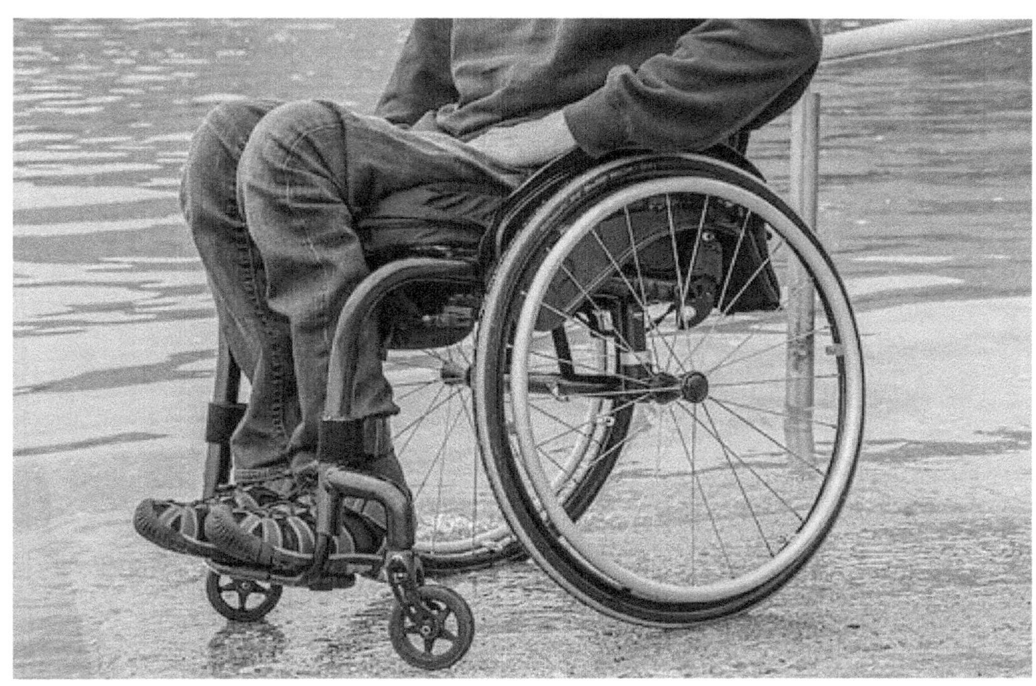

Most people with muscular dystrophy eventually lose their ability to **walk** and will need to use a wheelchair.

L is for Limb-Girdle

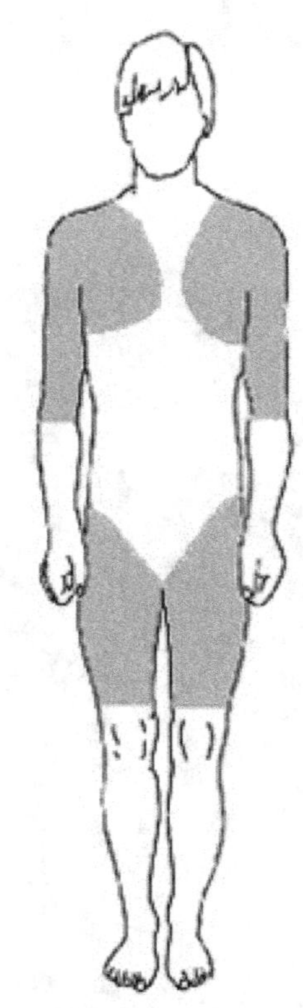

Limb-Girdle Muscular Dystrophy

-affects boys and girls equally

-progresses slowly

-mostly affects muscles in the pelvis, hips, shoulders, and back

-symptoms can appear at any age

M is for Myotonic

<u>Muscles Affected First</u>
Face, Arms, Neck, Hands,
Lower Legs, Hips

<u>Other Affected Areas</u>
Eyes, Throat, Skin, Nerves,
Heart, Stomach, Intestines

Myotonic Muscular Dystrophy causes problems with muscles being unable to relax. It affects more than 30,000 people in the U.S. There are 2 forms: Becker disease and Thomsen disease. It affects the muscles that are used for movement. The main symptom is stiff muscles.

N is for
Nine Types of
Muscular Dystrophy

There are **9 major types** of muscular dystrophy:

- o Becker
- o Congenital
- o Distal
- o Duchenne
- o Emery-Dreifuss
- o Facioscapulohumeral
- o Limb-girdle
- o Myotonic
- o Oculopharyngeal

O is for Occupational Therapy

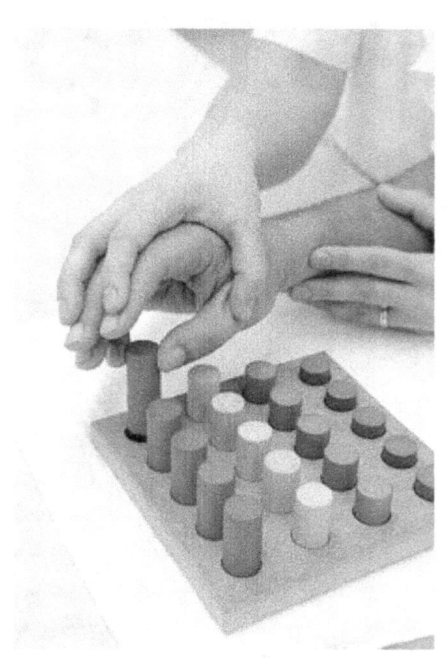

Occupational therapists help muscular dystrophy patients to do the activities that they need to do throughout a normal day. For example: getting dressed, brushing your hair, writing, etc. They can also teach you to use things like walkers and wheelchairs.

P is for Physical Therapy

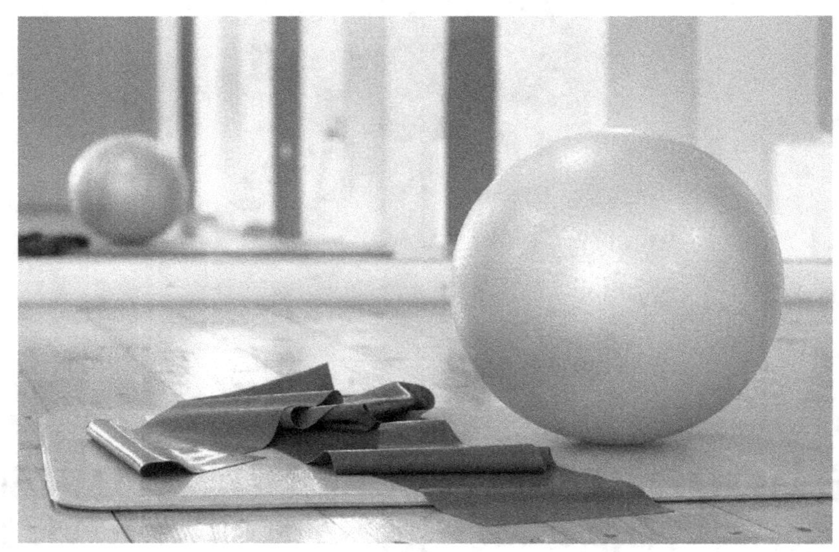

Physical therapists help muscular dystrophy patients to keep their joints and muscles as flexible as possible.

Q is for Quality of Life

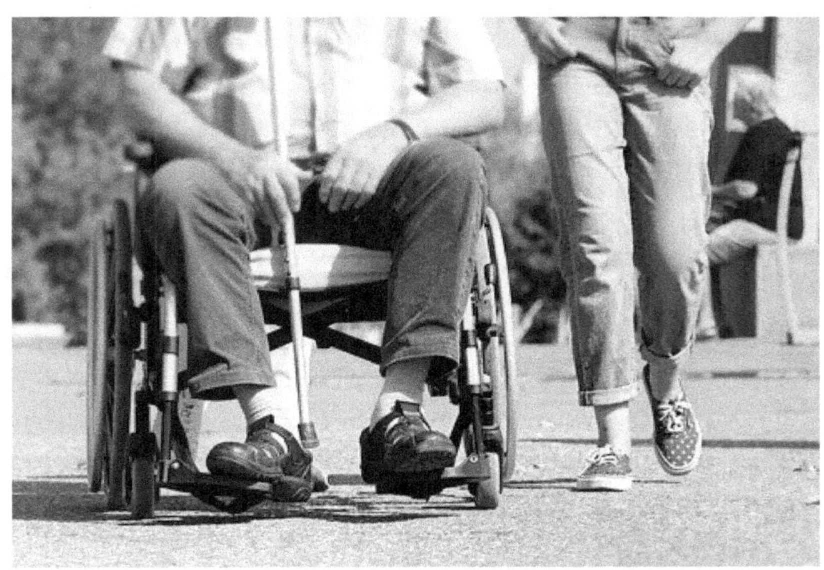

Right now, there is no way to cure or prevent muscular dystrophy. Muscle weakness can have an impact on a person's ability to do daily activities such as walking, breathing, swallowing, standing up, etc. Different types of therapy and medicine can improve a person's **quality of life**.

R is for Research

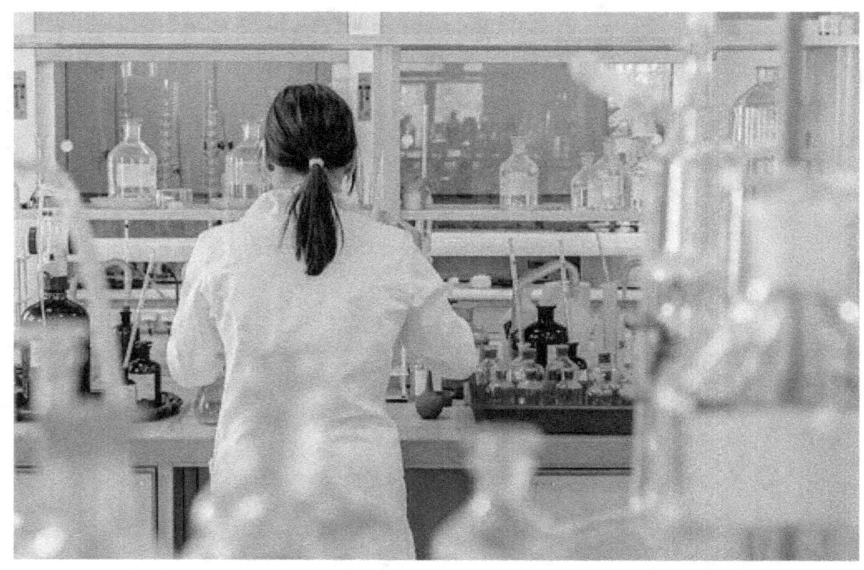

Since 1950, the Muscular Dystrophy Association (MDA) has invested more than $1 billion in **research**. Every year, the MDA supports hundreds of doctors and scientists researching new life-changing therapies for patients with muscular dystrophy. You can see information on their latest research at www.mda.org.

S is for Symptoms

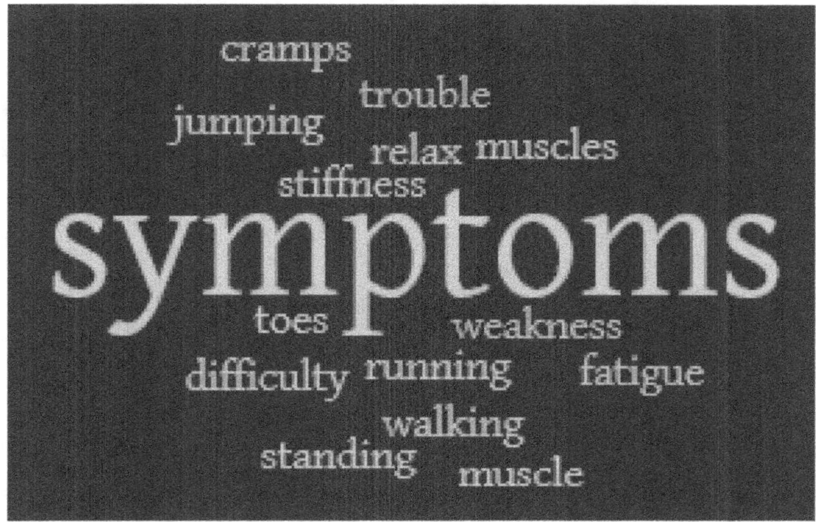

Different types of muscular dystrophy may result in the appearance of different **symptoms**. Some symptoms that may be experienced include:

-muscle weakness

-difficulty walking

-scoliosis

-walking on tip toe

-frequent falls

-trouble running or jumping

-difficulty getting up from lying down

T is for Treatment

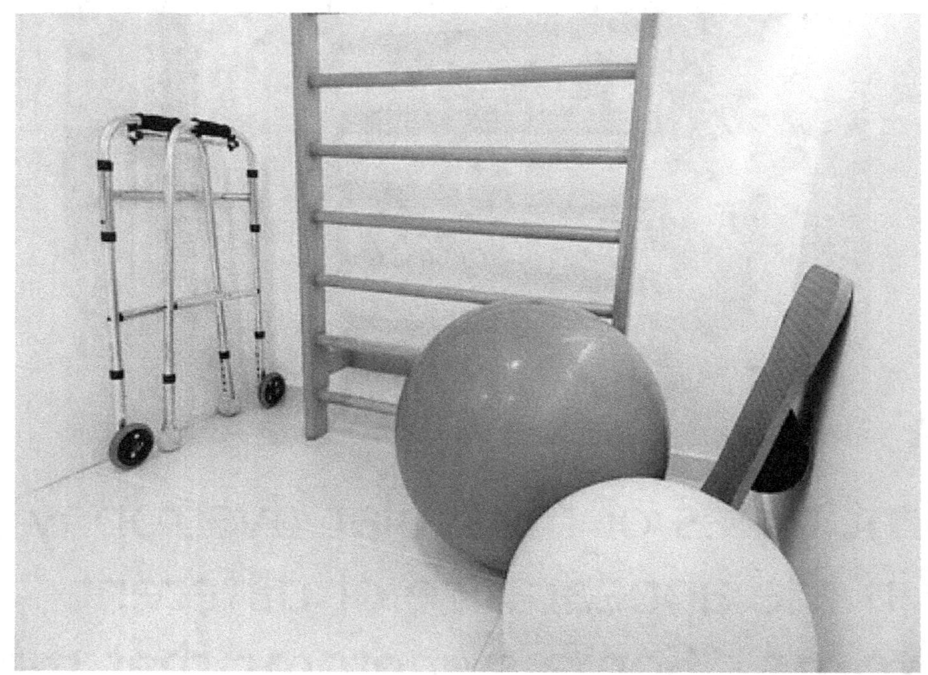

There is currently no cure for muscular dystrophy, but **treatment** can help a person with MD to live an active and independent life and remain mobile as long as possible. Treatments can include medication, occupational therapy, and physical therapy.

U is for Y-O-U!

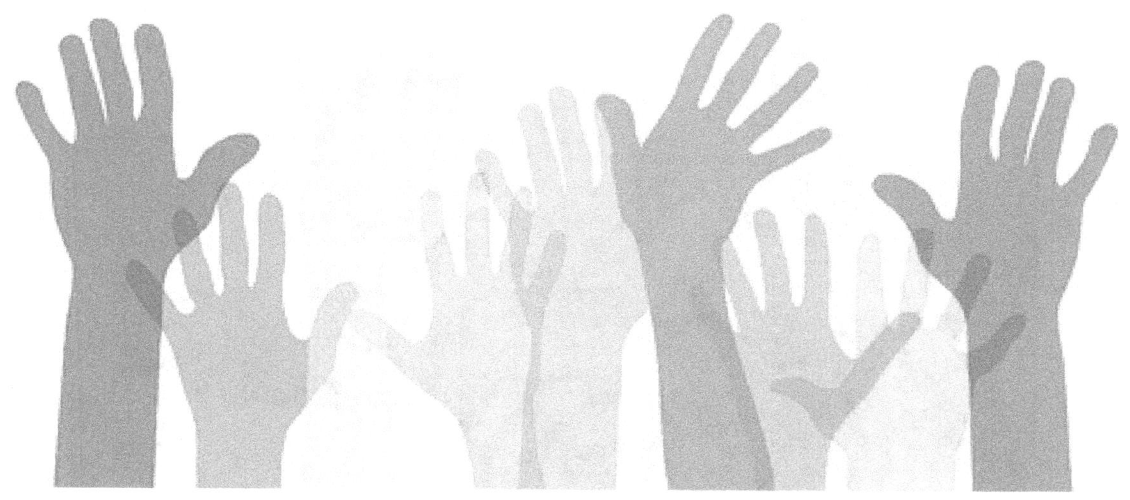

What can **YOU** do? Have a bake sale! Connect with people at your school and host a fundraiser! Contact your local Boy Scout or Girl Scout troop and work with them to raise money and to raise awareness! Look online for Muscular Dystrophy events that are happening in your area!

V is for Volunteer

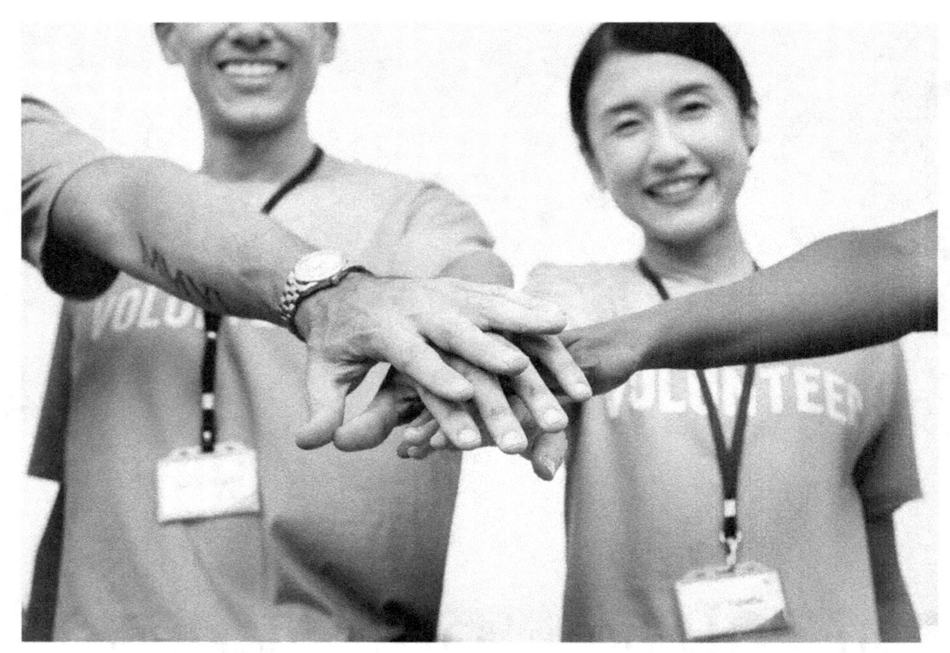

How can you help? You can **volunteer** to participate in a fundraiser or a walkathon for the Muscular Dystrophy Association where you live! You can help to raise money to help researchers to learn more about muscular dystrophy as they work to find a cure!

W is for Weakness

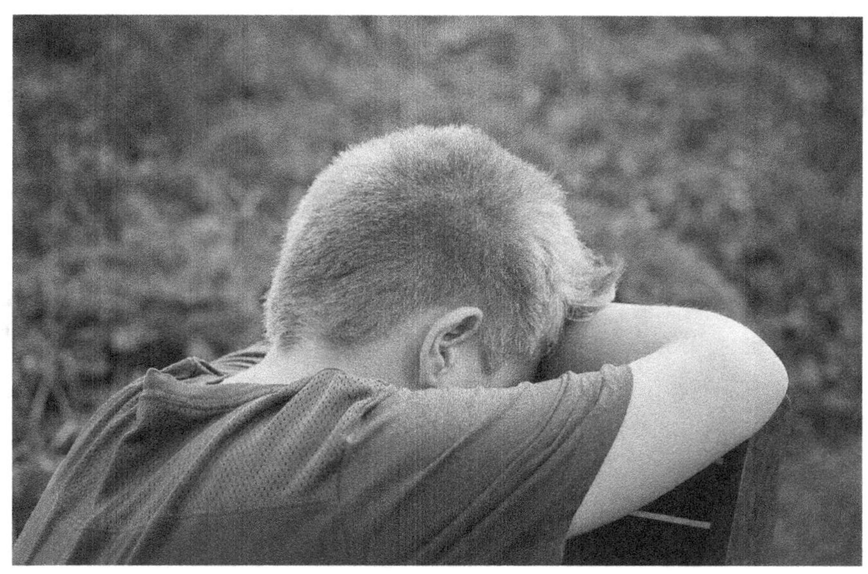

The **weakness** that people with muscular dystrophy feel is not the same as the weakness that you might feel after you finish running a long race. For someone with muscular dystrophy, that weakness is always there. Some types of muscular dystrophy cause our muscles to feel as weak as a baby or a toddler. Other types take longer for muscles to weaken...maybe as teenagers or adults.

X is for X-chromosome

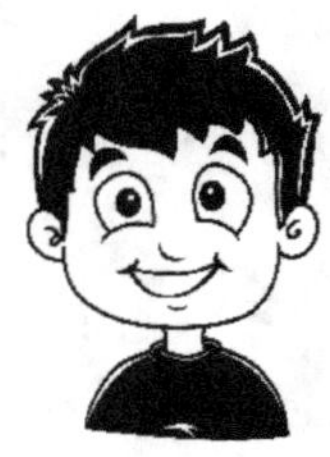

Dad does not have condition

X Y

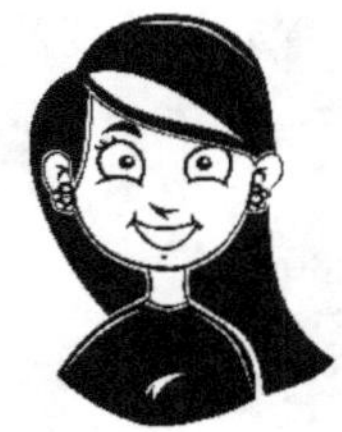

Mom is a carrier, does not have condition

X **X**

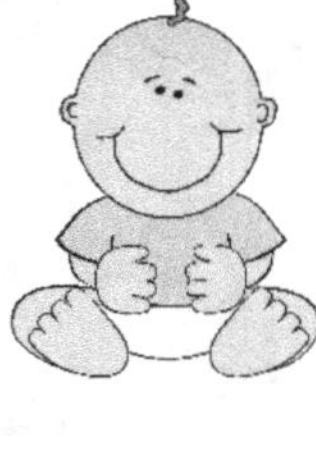

Son does not have condition

X Y

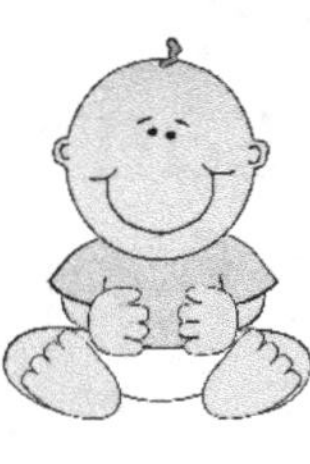

Son has condition

X Y

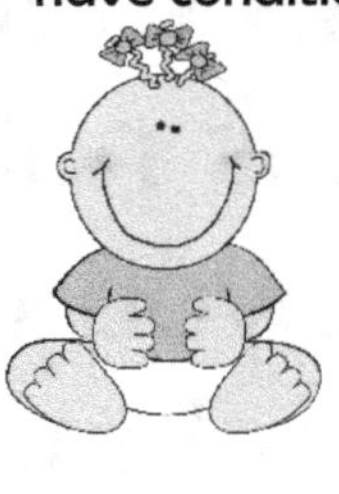

Daughter does not have condition

X X

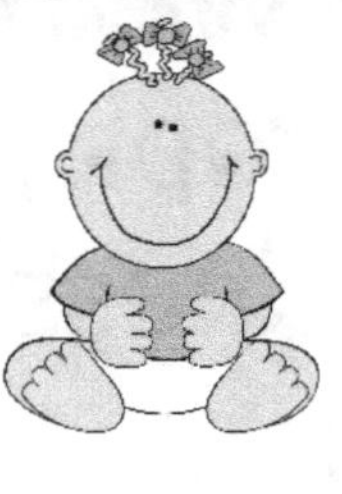

Daughter is a carrier, does not have condition

X **X**

Duchenne and Becker Muscular Dystrophy are inherited diseases. They are caused by mutations in the same gene on **the X-chromosome.**

Y is for Dystrophin

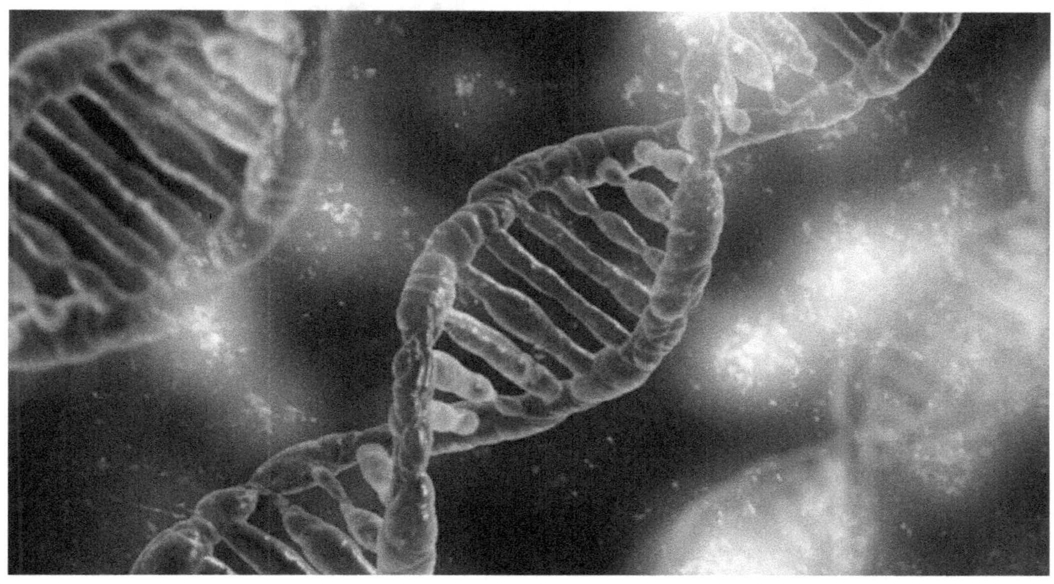

Dystrophin is a protein that is located in skeletal and cardiac muscles. It's job is to help stabilize and protect muscle fibers. Muscle cells without enough dystrophin become damaged over time. A lack of dystrophin leads to Duchenne MD. Not enough dystrophin, or poor quality dystrophin, leads to Becker MD.

Z is for Enzymes

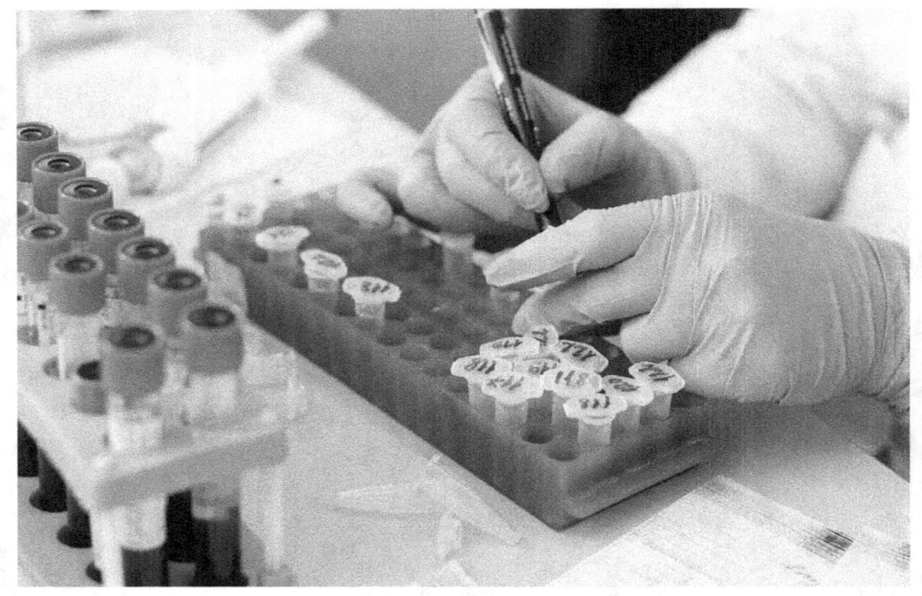

How can a doctor tell if someone has muscular dystrophy? Doctors can test for **enzymes** in the blood. Damaged muscles release enzymes into the blood, like creatine kinase. If doctors find a large amount of this enzyme in the blood, it can help the doctor to diagnose muscular dystrophy.